Intermittent Fasting Diet

Exclusive Guide For Losing Weight and Burning Fat in a Healthy Way.

The trademarks that are used are without any consent, and the publication of the trademark is without permission or backing by the trademark owner. All trademarks and brands within this book are for clarifying purposes only and are owned by the owners themselves, not affiliated with this document.

Contents

If you feel you have appreciated my effort, I kindly ask you to leave a (positive) review! It will help me to create something new and useful for your interest: =)

M.T.

PART 1

INTRODUCTION TO DIET AND INTERMITTENT FASTING

What is the diet?

In the field of nutrition, the term diet means the use of specific dietary habits for health or weight control reasons. A balanced diet is very important for normal physiological mechanisms of the body. While eating the right kinds of foods are important, it is also best to eat the right portions and quantities as well. This improves the immune system and health by following a healthy diet, but it will also assist with weight loss and control.

Carbohydrates, proteins, fats, vitamins, minerals, protein, and water are among the seven elements of a healthy diet. Among these seven elements, five are essential. We will discuss each element in detail.

There are many renowned methods of dieting. Few common tips which are very practical and have a great impact are listed below

1. The timing of meals is considered to be an essential aspect of any diet. The latest research indicates that new scheduling techniques, such as intermittent fasting or missing meals and taking pre-meal snacks, could be recommended as part of a larger lifestyle and dietary adjustment to eliminate cardiovascular risks.

2. Dieters who kept a daily calorie record lost twice as much weight as those who did not keep a calorie tracker, indicating that they are more mindful of what they eat and thus eat calculated calories if a person records his/her eating.

3. Water intake at regular intervals helps in weight management.

Our daily diets are made up of two essential types of nutrients, which are:

1. Macro-nutrients
2. Micronutrients

This is a universal classification for nutrients, and all subtypes of nutrients fall between them. Let's discuss these categories of nutrients in more detail.

Macro-nutrients:

As the name implies, macro-nutrients are larger and more diverse than the micro-nutrients. Nutrition in our daily food comes from our macro-nutrients, and they are essential to fulfill the basic energy needs of our bodies.

Macro-nutrients are subdivided into three classes:

1. Carbohydrates
2. Proteins
3. Fats

Carbohydrates:

Carbohydrates are an instant source of energy. All sugars fall under the category of carbohydrates. There are three subtypes of carbohydrates i.e

1. High glycemic
2. Medium glycemic
3. Low glycemic

Some nutritionists also divide these subclasses into very high and very low glycemic carbohydrates, but the standard classification comprises only the above-mentioned subtypes.

- High glycemic carbohydrates are those having a glycemic index of more than 70. High glycemic foods are notorious for increasing blood glucose levels very rapidly, and thus, these foods should be avoided. High glycemic foods are hazardous for diabetic patients. Processed white sugar is one example of high glycemic foods.
- Medium glycemic carbohydrates are those having a glycemic index between 56-69. These foods cannot increase blood glucose levels in a concise period of time. Banana is an example of medium glycemic food.
- Low glycemic carbohydrates have a glycemic index of less than 55, and these are the perfect choices for the ketogenic diet. These foods cannot shoot blood glucose

levels in a short period of time, and they are essential as a sustained source of energy. They release energy for an extended duration, but in small amounts, so they are perfect companions for those who are seeking to lose their extra pounds. Low glycemic carbohydrates are also very safe for diabetic patients. A true ketogenic diet contains less than 20 grams of carbohydrates in daily calorie intake, and these carbohydrates must be taken from low glycemic foods. Another benefit of using low glycemic food in the ketogenic diet is their stomach-filling capacity. These foods stall hunger and help in the prevention of over-eating habits. All green leafy vegetables and apples are examples of low glycemic foods.

Carbohydrates are an instant source of energy, and the simplest form of carbohydrates is glucose. Our body utilizes glucose as a principle energy-producing precursor. With the help of a ketogenic diet, a state of ketosis is achieved in which fats substitute glucose as the principal source of energy in the human body. An actual ketogenic diet comprises of very low amounts of carbohydrates (ideally from low glycemic foods). Less than 20 grams of carbohydrates are required daily in a real ketogenic diet, and this drastically reduced amount of carbohydrates helps in achieving ketosis.

The addition of green leafy vegetables helps in detoxifying the liver, kidneys, and other vital organs and prevent constipation. So it is a win-win situation to add low glycemic food to the diet. It is essential to know your current calorie count basal metabolic rates. It will help you to decide your carbohydrate intake. As a matter of fact, people with poor carbohydrate control must eat twenty grams of carbohydrates daily. People having reasonable carbohydrate control and an athletic lifestyle can eat fifty grams of carbs daily.

What are every human being's fundamental essentials? Nutrition, home, clothing, and accessories? And did you realize that the root of all these is carbohydrates? It would be fair to assume that life as we knew it would not survive on Earth without carbohydrates. Then let's learn about the chemical composition of carbohydrates somewhat more.

Carbohydrate is a class of carbonyl compounds (ketones) that occur naturally and also comprise multiple hydroxyl groups. This might also have byproducts that generate substances, likewise by the process of hydrolysis. They are indeed organic molecules which are most common in nature and are often referred to as "saccharides." The carbohydrates that are water-soluble and taste-sweet are named "sugars."

Protein:

Protein is the essential component of our diet, and our lean muscle mass needs the right amount of protein in the diet. The simplest unit of proteins is aminoacid. There are nearly twenty essential and non-essential amino acids in the human body. Essential amino acids cannot be formed within the body, and we have to consume them as a part of our diet, and non-essential amino acids can be made by our body during protein digestion. Protein in our diet must be used to replenish or increase the lean muscle mass, and it should never be used as a primary energy fuel of the body. When a person is starving, muscle glycogen is the first thing to be used as an energy source. If the person stays in starvation mode, stored fat in our body provides the vital energy, but if the starvation is prolonged enough, protein from our lean muscle mass is utilized as an emergency fuel. This is a dangerous scenario, and we need our lean muscle mass for the proper functioning of our body. Our lean muscle must never be utilized as an energy source, and that is why we consume a moderate amount of protein in the ketogenic diet to spare our muscles.

It is a common misconception that the ketogenic diet is bad for lean muscle mass as we don't eat high amounts of protein in the ketogenic diet. But it is just a myth as a real the ketogenic diet not only spares our lean muscle mass but in most cases, the ketogenic diet increases our lean muscle mass and decreases fat. It is again a win-win situation. Protein is available in meats, poultry, dairy, cereals, even in some fruits and vegetables. A ketogenic diet must be very low in carbohydrates, and we have to eat only those food sources which are enriched with good quality protein and very low carbohydrate content. All meats work great in the ketogenic diet as they are high in protein levels and contain almost zero carbohydrates. Eggs are also low carb proteinous food. Fruit, vegetables, cereals, and dairy products must be avoided in the ketogenic diet as they are high in carbohydrate levels.

Your required daily calories and BMR will help you in managing your daily protein intake. You can also find your daily protein levels by multiplying your lean muscle mass by 0.8. a person having a weight of 180 pounds with forty percent total body fat will have 108 pounds of lean muscle mass. An equation of 0.8x108 will give you the answer for your daily protein intake, and you will need almost 86 grams of protein per day.

In the ketogenic diet, protein makes up to 25% of total calories per day. It is noted that the ketogenic diet is not a high protein diet, so daily protein levels should be measured carefully.

Fats:

Fats are also called lipids, and the basic unit of fats is a fatty acid. Fats provide maximum energy, but they are not the principal source of energy in our body. The fundamental goal of a ketogenic diet is to achieve ketosis in our body, which is essential to shift our body's energy production from glucose to ketones. One gram of fat, when burnt, yields nine calories, which is more than double as provided by protein and carbohydrates. One gram of protein and carbohydrates will yield almost four calories.

Fats are subdivided into three types:

1. Trans-fats
2. Saturated fats
3. Unsaturated fats

Trans-fats are the most dangerous subtypes, and they are very hazardous to health. All deep-fried foods contain trans-fats. The fatty acids in these fats are distorted and damaged, so; these fats are of no use. We must avoid this type of fat at all costs, and it is the only prohibited subtype in the ketogenic diet.

All types of meat and dairy products are good sources of saturated fats. This type of fat is an essential precursor of all the hormones in our body. Human hormones are made up of cholesterol, and saturated fats provide essential concentrations of cholesterol. There was a terrible rep about saturated fats and cholesterol, but Dr. Atkins told the world about the benefits of fats. His words were not taken seriously, and he had to face a lot of criticism for what he said about fats. It is now well-established that all fats are not bad, and saturated fats are highly essential to produce our hormones. In many low-fat diets, saturated fats are removed from daily intake, and it disturbs the hormonal balance in the body. This is the reason behind low energy, bad moods, and fatigue in followers of the low-fat diet (especially saturated fat-free diet). The ketogenic diet makes sure to consume the right amounts of saturated fats.

Unsaturated fat:

These fats have chains of fatty acids combined with one or more double bonds, and most elite types of fats fall in this category. Unsaturated fats can be mono or polyunsaturated fats depending upon one or more double bonds, respectively. Unsaturated fats can be found in egg yolk, olive oil, and many foods of daily use. Polyunsaturated fats are mostly extracted from plant sources (such as olive oil). The right amount of unsaturated fats in our daily diet ensures better control of extra cholesterol in our bodies. Unsaturated fats help against stroke and heart attack.

In the ketogenic diet, we ensure to take nearly 70% calories from fats. Our daily fat intake can be broken down into 35% saturated fats, 35-40% monounsaturated fats, and 35-40% of polyunsaturated fats. This percentage ensures the inclusion of all-important fatty components in our daily diet. Fat acts as a lever in the ketogenic diet. In carb cycling and Atkins diet, carbohydrates are manipulated to ensure fat loss in our body, but in the ketogenic diet, carbohydrates and proteins remain constant for a prolonged period of time.

It is the fatty component of the ketogenic diet, which is manipulated to ensure the desired results.

In a neutral fat flux, your intake of dietary fat is perfectly balanced with fat burning (lipolysis). That means you are burning all the fats you have consumed, and it will maintain your body fat percentage.

In positive fat flux, your intake of dietary fat is more than the lipolysis. That means you are burning less fat than you have consumed. It will increase the body fat percentages in your body.

In negative fat flux, your daily intake of dietary fats is less than you burn. This is the real ketotic state, and more ketone bodies can be found in your blood. When the body burns all the fats taken from the daily diet, the next thing will be the consumption of fat from your stored adipose tissues. In negative fat flux, your overall body fat percentage will begin to decline. It is essential to achieve negative fat flux to ensure the constant burning of fat, which is stored as a cluster of fatty acids called the adipose tissues.

Micro-nutrients

This category of nutrients in our daily diet comprises of those salts, minerals, and vitamins which are present in food inherently, or we can take them as a supplement. Iron, magnesium, calcium, potassium, and vitamins are some examples. Some of them are required in trace amounts, yet they are essential for the proper regulation of the body's essential cycles.

Vitamins are available in fruits and green leafy vegetables. Eating plenty of raw fruits and vegetables can effectively target the daily requirements of many essential vitamins, which can help in the proper functioning of our muscles. Vitamin B12 is very important in the proper healing of our muscles, and it is present in green leafy vegetables (broccoli, Spinach, etc.) and also in carrots. Apple is also a great source of Vitamin B12. This vitamin is a special mention because lots of clinical research concluded that Vitamin B12 helps in preventing myofascial pain syndromes. Similarly, Vitamin C, Vitamin K, and other essential vitamins play important roles in optimized muscular performance. There are many vitamin brands available, but the best source of getting these vitamins is raw dietary food (vegetables and fruits).

Iron and potassium are the two most important minerals which are essential for the proper contraction of muscles. Iron is present in green leafy vegetables (especially in spinach), and banana is a great source of potassium.

Muscle cramps and trigger points are often caused by depleted calcium and vitamin D levels. Calcium is present in dairy products and eggs. Vitamin D can be taken as a dietary supplement, but sunlight is also a great source of Vitamin D.

Importance of proper water intake:
Our muscle is made up of protein, and when a muscle contracts, complex interactions occur between muscle fibers and filaments. These interactions are controlled by various minerals (calcium and potassium, and sodium), and proper homeostasis is essential to keep up the balance between these interactions. Homeostasis is the steady-state of the body in which every unit of our body acts in a precise manner. During a muscle activity, many enzymes are released, which control the complex interactions between muscle fibers. Creatine Kinase is the most important enzyme in muscles, which provides essential energy to muscles in the form of ATP.

These ATPs (adenosine triphosphates) are essential energy packets that are utilized when a muscle requires energy for its action. All of our enzymes work in the presence of water, and if our bodies are not hydrated enough, the actions of these enzymes cannot be accomplished. In a dehydrated state, creatine kinase cannot work properly, which leads to a severe energy crisis in our muscles. This, in turn, leads to severely painful muscle knots and muscle tightness. Moreover, a dehydrated muscle is not flexible enough, and it is very prone to injuries.

A healthy person should drink 3-4 liters of water daily. It is not only essential for muscles but also for our other crucial organs like the brain, heart, liver, stomach, etc. Dehydration leads to inflammation in our body, and toxic materials can slow the recovery of our muscles after a long hectic day.

WHAT IS INTERMITTENT FASTING?

Fasting, in reality, for so many, exists an article of faith. Some of the better-known examples are the Fasts of Lent, Yom Kippur, and Ramadan. For 180 days of the year, Greek Orthodox Christians are encouraged to fast ('Gluttony makes a man gloomy and afraid, but fasting makes him cheerful and brave,' according to Saint Nikolai of Zicha), while Buddhist monks fast on each lunar month's new moon and full moon.

Intermittent fasting is an eating pattern that cycles between fasting and eating times. It doesn't define which meals to consume, but when to eat them. It is not a diet in the traditional sense in this regard, but it is more accurately defined as a way of eating. Popular intermittent fasting strategies include fasting for 24 hours, twice a week, or fasting for 16 hours a day.

Uh, wait? Do you think that I do this every night already? Right... you do! You are still following the pattern of intermittent fasting, whether you knew it or not but to a limited extent if you wake up often during the night to eat. As a reader, you might have many questions in your mind, like skipping breakfast isn't bad for me? Why would anyone fast every day for 16 hours? What advantages are there? Behind this, is there any science, or are you really insane? Is that problematic? Slow down, readers. You will get answers to your every question one by one.

It is not about trying to deprive yourself of eating healthy, struggling to be impossibly slim, or cheating yourself not to be a food lover. A healthy diet comprises carbohydrates, proteins, fat, vitamins, and minerals in the appropriate quantities is the right way to do it.

IF has been around in different ways for years as a weight-loss strategy, but was widely popularized in 2012 by BBC journalist Dr. Michael Mosley's TV documentary Eat Easy, Live Longer and book The Fast Diet, followed by the book the 5:2 Diet based on her own experience by journalist Kate Harrison, and subsequently, by Dr. Jason Fung's 2016 bestseller The Obesity Code as stories of its efficacy gained popularity IF produced steady positive fame. The ancient Greeks claimed that fasting improves intellectual capabilities.

Only think about the last time you enjoyed a big Thanksgiving meal. Did you feel more productive and mentally alert afterward? Or did you, instead, feel drained and perhaps a little loopy? The latter is more probable. Blood is funneled into the digestive tract to deal with the tremendous influx of nutrition, allowing less blood going to the brain. Intermittent fasting is able to bring us back into contact with our human self. It is a path not just to weight loss but also to health and well-being in the coming years. Researchers are only now beginning to discover and show how effective it can be a method.

Most importantly, without going on an insane diet or limiting your calories to nil, it's a perfect way to become lean. Actually, most of the time, when you begin intermittent fasting, you'll try to keep your calories the same. (During a shorter period, most people eat larger meals.) In addition, intermittent fasting is a healthy way to preserve muscle mass when being lean. The predominant reason that people are seeking intermittent fasting is to lose weight. I'll talk about how intermittent fasting results in fat loss.

One question will also raise in your mind that what should I eat? Eat high-fiber foods during your eating periods such as nuts, beans, vegetables, and fruits and protein-rich foods like beef, fish, poultry, or nuts. Only drink plenty of water. Water plays a very important role in fat burning.

Your body has been built for fasting. At a time when food was scarce, we have evolved; we are the result of millennia of feasting and famine. The reason we adapt so well to Intermittent Fasting is that it mimics the world in which modern humans were shaped, even more accurately than three meals a day. Intermittent fasting is able to bring us back into contact with our human self. It is a path not only to weight loss but also to health and well-being in the long term. Scientists are only now starting to discover and show how effective it can be as a weapon. There are several ways of Intermittent Fasting that are different. For 24 hours or longer, others require eating nothing. Others provide, once a day, every other day, a single low-calorie meal. I tried both, but on a daily basis, I could not imagine doing either. It was simply too hard, I found. Later, will discuss it.

We know that traditional diet advice actually doesn't work for several people. A radical alternative is a 1-Easy Diet. It has the power to alter the way we think of weight loss and food.

2-The Fast Diet demands that we not only care about what we consume but when we eat it.

3-No complex rules need to be followed; the strategy is versatile, understandable, and user-friendly.

4-There is no everyday slog of calorie control-no exhaustion, dissatisfaction, or serial deprivation that determines traditional diet plans.

5-Yeah, it includes fasting, but not as you know it; you're not going to die on any given day.

6-The foods you love can always be enjoyed. The bulk of the time.

7-Sticking to the basic program would ensure that it stays off until the weight is off.

8- Just one advantage of the Fast Diet is weight loss. The true dividend is the future long-term health benefits that reduce your risk of a variety of diseases, including diabetes, heart disease, and cancer.

9-You will eventually come to learn that it is not just a diet. It is even more than that: it is a plan for a balanced, long life that is sustainable.

This fasting will help lower cholesterol, boost glucose regulation, decrease liver fat, and improve blood pressure, in addition to lower body weight. Patients inform me that they have enhanced stamina, better muscle control, and sleep quality.

Help in weight loss:

To go on a lengthy fast will be one way to lose weight. As a weight loss regime, I would not suggest it because it is absolutely unsustainable. If they pair it with a rigorous workout regime, muscle and fat are lost by people who go on extended fasts. Then, as they would inevitably do when they stop, the danger is that they will add the weight right back on.

Fasting of Alternate-Day:

Alternate Day Fasting is one of the most widely researched ways of short-term fasting (ADF). As the name suggests, it means that every other day you get no food or very little food. Dr. Krista Varady of the University of Illinois at Chicago is one of the few researchers to have done human studies in this field. A lot of ADF research, shocked with the result that people don't go wild on their feeding days, except though they're allowed to. Researches figured that people would eat 175 percent the next day; they would only adjust entirely and lose no weight. Most people, though, consume around 110%, just slightly above what they normally eat. Researchers think that it includes the size of the stomach, how much it can extend. And it's actually very hard to consume nearly twice the amount of food you usually eat. Over time, you can do it; fat people, their stomachs get bigger to handle, you know, 5000 calories a day. But it's actually pretty hard just to do it right.

The researchers and participants had believed that more weight would be lost by people on the low-fat diets than those on the high-fat diet. But it was the other way around, if anything. The participants lost an average of kg on the high-fat diets, and those on the low-fat diet lost 4.2kg. They both dropped about 7 cm around their waists.

He assumes that compliance was the key reason why this happened. The participants randomized to the high-fat diets were much more likely to stick to it mainly because they found it a lot more appealing than those on the low-fat diets. And it wasn't weight loss alone. Impressive reductions in LDL cholesterol, poor cholesterol, and blood pressure were seen in both groups. This meant that their risk of cardiovascular disease, heart attack, or stroke was decreased. Another essential advantage to intermittent fasting is that you don't appear to sacrifice the muscle you might lose in a standard calorie-restricted regime.

The two-day fasting:

One of the issues with ADF, which is why I'm not so keen on it, is that every other day you have to do it. In my experience, this can be both socially awkward and mentally taxing. Your week has no routine, and other people, friends, and relatives find it difficult to keep track of what your days of fasting and feeding are. To start with, I was not especially overweight, but I was not concerned about losing too much weight too fast. A variety of studies have been performed testing the impact of a two-day fast on female volunteers. Researchers have divided 115 women into three classes in a recent survey. One participant group was instructed to adhere to a Mediterranean diet of 1500 calories and was also urged to avoid high-fat foods and alcohol. Another participant group was instructed to eat five days a week normally, but on the other two days to eat a 650-calorie, low carb diet.

PART 2

THE SCIENCE OF INTERMITTENT FASTING

Digestion, Hormones, and How Food Is Stored for Energy

The second that food enters your mouth, your body begins the hard work of turning that food into cellular energy. However, the path isn't always easy or straightforward, and if you eat the wrong foods or consume them in excess, your body may develop problems.

The body's endocrine system includes a vast network of glands that release hormones into the bloodstream to regulate all the body's functions, including sleep, metabolism (the conversion of food to energy for cell function), reproduction and sex drive, mood, hunger, and more. When we eat, the pancreas—a narrow, six-inch-long organ that sits behind the stomach and is part of both the endocrine and digestive systems—secretes the hormone insulin. Insulin signals to the rest of the body that food is now available to process into energy, and this food energy (calories) needs to be stored away for the future.

The body stores food energy in two different ways: sugar and body fat. Sugar is available for quick energy, while fat is kept in reserve, available to burn when our body doesn't have blood sugar at the ready. Let's talk about sugar first, as the stable regulation of blood sugar—also known as glucose—is one of the central benefits of fasting.

One of the easiest ways to spike your blood sugar is to eat carbohydrates, which, chemically speaking, are chains of sugars. When we eat carbohydrates, some of this sugar is used by cells in the kidneys, liver, brain, and more. If there are carbs left over, they're stored in the liver as glycogen, another chain of sugar. We'll come back to glycogen in just a minute.

The other way our body stores energy is body fat. When we eat dietary fat (found in all kinds of plant and animal foods, from potato chips to red meat to milk), the individual fat molecules, called triglycerides, are absorbed directly into the bloodstream and delivered to fat cells. If we eat too much glucose and exceed the body's ability to store it in the liver as glycogen, the liver converts this glucose to triglycerides. The triglycerides then feed fat cells.

These two systems of energy storage—glycogen and fat—are complementary. Glycogen is easy to use and simple for the liver to process, but the liver has limited space to store it. Body fat is harder to get to and more difficult for the liver to break down, but it offers the advantage of unlimited storage space (as anyone worried about the rolls of fat on their belly knows all too well!). Think of glycogen as a refrigerator. You can easily put food into it and take it out at a moment's notice, but you only have so many shelves. Think of body fat like a deep basement freezer. It's harder to get to, harder to cook the food in it (because it's frozen), but it's huge and almost never full.

Insulin and the Development of Diabetes

As I stated previously, insulin is the hormone that signals your body when it's time to convert food into energy. But its job doesn't stop there. Insulin also regulates the body's glucose levels, making sure they don't spike or plummet. It does so by helping to extract glucose from the blood to store it in the liver as glycogen or in the body as fat. Because the body needs fat for protection, warmth, and energy in times of famine, insulin also prevents us from using too much body fat as a source of energy.

If your insulin levels are high, the body will put food energy into storage, both in the fridge and the freezer. Problems begin, however, when your pancreas goes into overdrive, secreting too much insulin. How does this happen? All foods, which contain a variety of macronutrients (protein, fat, and carbohydrates), will stimulate insulin production to some degree, but certain foods are more effective than others. The worst offenders in this regard are refined carbohydrates, like white bread, sugary drinks, cakes, and cookies.

If we eat lots of sugar or carbohydrate-rich foods too often, as is the case with the typical Western diet, where people regularly eat six or seven carb-heavy meals or snacks a day, our insulin levels will spike. High levels of insulin tell the body to keep trying to store food energy, preventing us from burning our fat stores. We are, in essence, continuing to restock the refrigerator while wondering why our basement freezer is bursting at the seams.

Eventually, when there is too much insulin flooding your system, the cells in your pancreas that produce it can no longer respond, and your blood glucose levels become high. If they *stay* high, you can now call yourself one of the estimated 500 million people in the world with type 2 diabetes.

Measuring and Treating Diabetes

If you develop diabetes, your symptoms may include increased thirst, fatigue, blurred vision, hunger even though you're eating more than you normally do, frequent urination, tingling, pain or numbness in your hands or feet, or cuts or bruises that are slow to heal. But you may not have *any* symptoms. Many people discover they're at risk of diabetes or already have it only after they have a blood test.

There are several tests doctors use to determine if a person has diabetes, but I'll talk about two of them because many of my clients have them regularly—and many see their results improve dramatically after they try fasting.

The first test is the A1c test. This simple blood test measures what percentage of your hemoglobin—a protein in red blood cells that carries oxygen—is covered with sugar. A1c measures average blood sugar levels over two to three months, so one carb-heavy meal won't necessarily impact the results. People without diabetes have low A1c levels, between 4 percent and 5.6 percent. If your A1c levels are between 5.7 percent and 6.4 percent, you're at risk for developing diabetes, often referred to as prediabetic. And if your levels are over 6.5 percent, you have type 2 diabetes.

The other test is called the fasting plasma glucose test, or FPG. This test measures blood glucose levels at one point in time, and it's given after you've fasted for eight hours, typically in the morning. A high result—indicating you have diabetes—is anything over a level of 126 mg/dL. A prediabetic level is between 100 and 125 mg/dL, and anything under 100 mg/dL is considered normal.

If your test results are in the prediabetic range, you'll need to adjust the foods you eat and perhaps consider some of the medications I'll discuss below. But remember to focus your health efforts not just on diabetes. Midrange A1c or fasting glucose levels also mean you're at risk for heart disease, stroke, cognitive difficulties, or insulin resistance (a disease in which your body doesn't respond well to insulin and raises your blood sugar).

In addition to weight loss, exercise, and diet modifications—typically a diet low in sugar and carbs—the most common treatment for diabetes is a prescription medication. Metformin is the gateway drug for diabetes treatment, and it works by limiting the amount of glycogen your liver converts into glucose, as well as helping your body use insulin more productively. Other drugs—including sulphonylureas—help the body produce more insulin or become more sensitive to it, excrete glucose into the urine, or slow digestion. Typically, the last resort for diabetes treatment is insulin, given by subcutaneous injection.

However, it's disheartening—to say the least—that fasting is not recommended by the health community. Why? Because more than any drug or diet modification, fasting helps control your insulin. Type 2 diabetes is essentially a disease of too much sugar and too much insulin. What decreases sugar and insulin? Fasting. When your insulin is in check, your blood sugar stays in check, your weight stabilizes or decreases, and your risk of developing any number of chronic health conditions goes down.

Where Fasting Comes In

If I could sum up fasting in one sentence, I would say this: fasting regulates your hormones. It's more than a diet; it resets your body's internal controls, allowing it to burn the right amount of energy to keep you alive.

When we don't eat (fast), insulin levels fall, and this signals our body that no more food is available. In order to survive, the cells then draw upon the stored energy supply, either in the form of glycogen or, if that's been fully expended, fat. This is the reason we don't die in our sleep every night, or why we can live a few hours—or a few days or more—without eating. The body has a wondrous ability to store food energy, then find it in either the refrigerator or freezer to burn it.

Therefore, it figures that the most logical solution to keeping our blood sugar levels stable, allowing the body to continue to use its stored reserves of energy, is to fast. By not eating, we allow insulin levels to drop, which tells the body that food is no longer available and that it's time to eat some of the food in the fridge (glycogen) or freezer (body fat). Weight loss and preventing type 2 diabetes—as well as a host of chronic conditions I'll outline in the next chapter—are about correcting the underlying hormonal imbalance that caused obesity. This hormonal imbalance, again, is an insulin level that stays high for too long.

Fasting and Metabolism

But what about metabolism? Doesn't fasting kill it, as many of you have heard? For that matter, what *is* metabolism? Our metabolism, or basal metabolic rate (BMR), is the amount of energy (calories) required to keep our bodies alive while we are at rest. BMR is the measure of what we need to keep our body's very basic functions—such as brain activity, circulation, and digestion—chugging along. If you have a high metabolism, your body burns energy more efficiently, and you tend not to put on weight rapidly. If it's lower, weight loss will be more of a struggle.

Our BMR is not fixed. Our bodies may increase or decrease BMR by 30 to 40 percent, depending on our diets, level of activity, age, body temperature, and more. But, from a dietary perspective, the most significant determinant of BMR is insulin.

The body only exists in one of two states: the "fed" state, after we've eaten, and the "fasted" state when we have not eaten. In the fed state, insulin levels are high, and the body wants to store food energy as sugar or fat. Our metabolism is humming. In the fasted state, when insulin levels are low, the body wants to burn stored food energy. So, we're either storing calories or burning calories, but not both at the same time.

If we elevate insulin levels (by eating foods that stimulate insulin) and keep them persistently high (by constantly eating—say, by consuming six or seven snacks or meals per day instead of three), then the body must stay in the "fed" state. The body stores calories because those are the instructions we've given it. If all the calories are going into storage, then there are fewer calories to use, and therefore the body must slow down its energy expenditure, or BMR.

Suppose we are eating 2,000 calories per day and burning 2,000 calories per day. We neither gain nor lose body fat. We now reduce our calories to 1,500 by eating high-carb, low-fat foods six or seven times per day, as many health professionals urge us to do. Insulin levels stay high, but calories drop. Now, the body cannot burn body fat stores because insulin is high, and we are in the "fed" state. With only 1,500 calories coming in, the body must reduce its calorie expenditure to 1,500 as well. We cannot make up this caloric deficit because insulin prevents us from burning fat. We are in "fat storage" mode. This is the dirty little secret of the low-fat diet. At first, the weight comes off, but as our BMR drops, the weight plateaus and then eventually returns.

What happens during fasting? A study of four consecutive days of fasting—that is, four full days without any food to eat—showed that BMR increases by about 10 percent. Yes, the metabolic rate increases when you don't eat. Why? We know that fasting decreases insulin but increases counter-regulatory hormones, so-called because they run counter to insulin. If insulin falls, these hormones go up. If insulin rises, these hormones go down. The counter-regulatory hormones include noradrenaline (responsible for stimulating muscle contraction and heart rate), growth hormone (stimulates cell growth and regeneration), and cortisol (the so-called stress hormone, responsible for triggering motivation and action). If noradrenaline increases, then the metabolic rate is also expected to go up.

The increase in BMR is likely a survival response. Imagine that you are a caveman. It's winter, and there is nothing to eat. If your metabolic rate decreases, that means that for every day you do not eat, you get a little weaker. This makes it that much harder to find and hunt for food. It's a vicious death spiral. As you get weaker, you'll be less likely to find food. As you don't find food, you get weaker. If this is what happens to your body, you would not have survived. Your body is just not that stupid.

Instead, your body switches fuel sources. Instead of relying on food, you turn to stored food (body fat), and your body does not shut down. It ramps up by increasing noradrenaline, cortisol, and the other counter-regulatory hormones. You power up by using a different fuel source. Concentration increases. Focus increases. So BMR increases during fasting. If you maintain BMR during weight loss, as opposed to burning 500 calories less per day, that is a huge advantage.

So, the key to the energy balance equation of "Calories In, Calories Out" is not the number of calories we eat and the exercise we do. That is virtually irrelevant. The key is to control hunger and maintain basal metabolic rate. In order to do that, we must eat foods that increase satiety hormones and keep insulin (fat-storing hormone) low. Fasting provides the hormonal changes necessary to lose weight in the long term success. Hunger decreases while BMR is maintained. And guess what? Fasting has been used for thousands of years, during which time obesity has been no more than a passing footnote in the pantheon of human illness.

PART 3

AMAZING IMPACTS OF INTERMITTENT FASTING

Fasting and Your Brain

The brain is a remarkable, complex, and resilient organ, and it's one that's not impacted negatively by fasting. So, if you're concerned that fasting will cause you to be mentally slow, dull, or foggy, worry no more.

Fasting may even *help* your brain. I say "may" because, unfortunately, no authoritative studies exist on fasting's impact on the brain. However, two human studies—one that measured brain activity after a twenty-four-hour fast and one that measured it after two days—established that reaction time, memory, mood, and general function were not impaired by fasting. And in a study of rats who were put on a fast, the mammals improved their scores of motor coordination, cognition, learning, and memory. In addition, they showed increased brain connectivity and new neuron growth. Now, I know rats aren't humans, but these results echo what so many of my clients say: that fasting makes them feel sharper.

Evolution also provides some clues to how fasting can help your brain. During times of severe caloric restriction, the organs of many mammals shrink in order to survive. But there are two exceptions: the brain and the male testicles. Obviously, the testicles stay the same size so that the males of the species can continue to attempt to mate, but what about the brain? Think about how you'd feel if you were starving. You'd want to be sharp and focused so you could search for food, right? That's what happens with most mammals. Conversely, when we eat too much, we may experience brain fog, or what's often known as "food coma." Consider how you feel after a huge Thanksgiving dinner: lethargic, dull, and able to focus only on the thought of a nap.

The most encouraging research I've seen is the animal studies that demonstrate that rats who were subjected to fasts showed fewer symptoms in models of Alzheimer's, Huntington's, and Parkinson's disease. Fasting induces autophagy—a cellular process that helps the body clear out old or damaged cell parts—and, in these studies, rats on a fast saw a decrease in the accumulated proteins that are a hallmark of Alzheimer's. Imagine if fasting could prevent, treat, or even reverse these heartbreaking degenerative neurological conditions? Lives could be saved, suffering reduced, and we'd save tens of billions of dollars in healthcare costs.

Fasting and Cancer

Cancer is the second-leading cause of death worldwide, killing about 10 million people every year. One out of six people will die from it. Many cancers develop due to genetic factors, unintended toxic exposure, viruses, or some other, often unknown cause. For the most part, these unfortunate cases are difficult to prevent. But there are promising studies that show that cancers that were previously thought to be unavoidable may be preventable, in part, through fasting.

One of the keys to these findings, as with type 2 diabetes and obesity, is insulin. If you extract breast cancer cells from tissue, it's quite simple to grow them in a lab. If you add glucose, epidermal growth factor (EGF), and insulin, they multiply rapidly. If you then take away the insulin, they die. Let me repeat that: breast cancer cells proliferate with high levels of insulin and die without it. What lowers insulin levels? Fasting.

The second reversible link to cancer is obesity. A 2003 study released by the American Cancer Society highlighted the findings from 900,000 US men and women. From 1982 to 1998, these people were tracked every few years to determine who had died and how they'd died. At each interval, their BMI (body mass index) was also factored in. While all were free from cancer at the start of the study, after sixteen years, just over 57,000 of them were dead from cancer. Shockingly, for those with a BMI over 40, the death rates from all cancers combined were 52 percent higher for men and 62 percent higher for women. BMI was positively associated with death from esophageal, colon, rectal, liver, gallbladder, pancreatic, kidney, non-Hodgkin's lymphoma, multiple myeloma, breast, stomach, prostate, cervical, uterine, and ovarian cancers. Researchers concluded that being overweight or obese accounts for 14 percent of all deaths from cancer in men and 20 percent for women. The evidence was clear: obesity is a major risk factor for cancer. What helps you lose weight? Fasting.

Finally, autophagy may slow down cancerous growths or prevent cancer from occurring—a finding that shocked scientists, who had previously believed that autophagy *increased* cancer growth. A 2019 study published in *Nature* concluded that autophagy played a major role in killing certain cells linked to cancer. When autophagy is stopped, these harmful cells can continue to replicate, fueling the growth of cancer. What causes autophagy? Once again, fasting.

Fasting and Metabolic Syndrome

Metabolic syndrome, also called Syndrome X, is a group of conditions that meet three of the following five criteria: abdominal obesity (as measured by waist circumference), hyperglycemia (type 2 diabetes), high triglycerides, low HDL, and hypertension.

The common factor among these conditions is that they all involve an excess of insulin. When insulin is too high for too long, the body stores more body fat than it needs to. Cells become overloaded with glucose, and they become resistant to insulin. Glucose from the blood can no longer go into the cells, and blood glucose levels become elevated. This is the disease known as type 2 diabetes. When the liver is overloaded with glucose, excess sugar gets stored as fat, and fatty liver develops. Attempting to unload all this extra fat, the liver exports the glucose into the blood, which causes blood triglyceride levels to increase and HDL levels to decrease. In short, excess insulin causes a series of problems that collapse, one by one, like dominoes.

Since metabolic syndrome is a disease of too much insulin, lowering insulin levels is critical to reversing it. Refined carbohydrates cause the greatest increase in insulin, so eating a diet low in refined carbs and sugar is a great start. Because all foods contain a mix of protein, carbohydrates, and fat, eating even those foods that are healthy will raise your insulin level somewhat. This is why fasting is so effective for treating metabolic syndrome. When you refrain from eating, your insulin levels drop and remain at a lower baseline. Clearly, fasting helps to stabilize blood sugar. But having stable blood sugar levels is only one of many benefits of a fasting lifestyle. As we will soon see, it can do wonders for the mind as well as the body.

If you feel you have appreciated my effort, I kindly ask you to leave a (positive) review! It will help me to create something new and useful for your interest: =)

M.T.

PART 4
THINGS REQUIRED TO START INTERMITTENT FASTING

You are at the beginning of an exciting journey. You may be tense and eager, ready for the gun to fire so you can launch toward the challenge. Or—if you're like most of us who've battled weight and health challenges for years—you might be anxious about what lies ahead.

Desperation and self-doubt are some of my most familiar companions. They sit next to me, invisible to the rest of the world, whispering words of discouragement softly into my ear. They remind me that I have failed at eating better and getting healthier for most of my adult life. They snicker at my hope and laugh at my thoughts that this time might be different. Self-doubt nags at me, asking: *Why would I ever think I can fast if I haven't been able to stop shoveling massive amounts of food into my mouth for decades?*

It's time to stop thinking this way. No matter how many calorie-restriction diet plans you've tried in the past . . . yes, you can do this.

Remember: you are not the problem. You've simply been fed incorrect information for years. But with the right knowledge, your body can heal itself. In fact, it may be even easier than you think because it's possible your body and mind are not as broken as you suspect. Like me, you may discover that beneath the extra weight, you are healthier than you could ever imagine. This is why a plethora of people who fast heal their type 2 diabetes, resolve their high blood pressure or go off their medications with shocking speed. My father is a case in point.

Lies We've All Heard About Fasting

- **FASTING WILL MAKE YOU SICK.** Quite the opposite! Fasting can lower your risk of heart disease, cancer, type 2 diabetes, and high blood pressure.

- **FASTING WILL CAUSE YOUR BLOOD SUGAR TO CRASH.** Your body does a wonderful job regulating blood sugar levels, so there's little chance of your body having a negative hypoglycemic response.

- **FASTING WILL SLOW DOWN YOUR METABOLISM.** There is no research that shows that fasting—even fasts up to three days—suppresses metabolic rates.

- **YOU'LL DIE OF HUNGER.** This is my favorite! Have you ever skipped a meal? Look what happened! You didn't die. I know this because you are reading this book.

Goals Start with You

If you are out of the habit of goal setting, it is time to get back in the groove.

Many people feel comfortable putting everyone else in their lives first when it comes to setting goals. They make a goal that their sixth graders will get on the honor roll this semester or that their spouse will get a raise by the end of the year. When did we get so busy helping others that we forgot to take a moment to consider what *we* truly desire?

Now is the time for *you*. You are reading this book to discover how your body, mind, and life can be changed when you incorporate fasting. Start by deciding what you want to gain by fasting. The answer can be anything at all.

Your goal is individual to your wants and needs—and it is vitally important to your success. Reaching your goal may not be fast or stress-free, but nothing worthwhile ever comes easily. Picture your fasting skills as a muscle you must exercise, rest, and grow. Some days you'll flex that muscle with ease. Other days are going to be a challenge. It's during those times that focusing on your goal becomes important. When you've had a few difficult days in a row and find yourself wondering, *Is this worth it?* It's your goal that will remind you why you are on this journey—and that *you* are worth it.

Goals Change

This road can get bumpy sometimes, so I want you to create one very specific goal—or, if you must, no more than two—that will help keep you motivated. I'm sure you want to achieve many things, but limiting your focus to the one or two most important goals will help you keep your eye on the prize and lessen your chances of getting overwhelmed. The amazing thing is that once you accomplish just a few small goals, you'll find that some of your other hopes start to come to fruition, too. For example, maybe your goal was to go from an A1c level of 7 percent (diabetic) to 6 percent (prediabetic). One of the unexpected side benefits could be that the tingling in your toes—which had been a constant nuisance—stops. Or that, suddenly, you're able to walk up a flight of stairs without losing your breath. Your goals should be clear, specific, concrete. For example, an unclear goal would be "I want to be more active" (active how and when?), while a clear goal could be "I want to walk a 5k."

Some goals to guide you:

- Get off type 2 diabetes medicine
- Wear a new dress for my high school reunion
- Complete a triathlon
- Reduce my body fat percentage
- Buy pants that aren't stretchy
- Get pregnant
- Get sick less often
- Get off blood pressure medicine
- Wear high heels that don't come in a wide size
- Be able to walk with the dog one mile
- Stop having migraines
- Have better focus at work
- Play with my grandkids
- Lose a certain number of pounds

Once you're clear about what your goals are, I want you to write them down in three places. You can keep your goals on a piece of paper in your top desk drawer at work, scribble them on your mirror at home, type them into your phone, or make them your computer screensaver. Every time you come across your list, read it out loud three times, adding the words "I will" at the beginning of each goal. You can also say them silently in your head.

So often, we put aside what we want for "just one more day" until the "one more day" stretches into months and years. Keeping your goals in the front of your mind and reminding yourself of them daily will help reinforce them.

What Motivates You?

There are two types of motivation: intrinsic and extrinsic. Intrinsic motivation means that what drives a person comes from within and that their desire to perform a specific task is in accordance with their belief system. Eve's desire to "get hot" and "feel hot" is an example of intrinsic motivation. Other examples would be to feel better, have more energy, and reduce your risk of type 2 diabetes.

In extrinsic motivation, an individual's stimulus is external, even though the results will still benefit the individual. A classic example of extrinsic motivation is money. In this case, that might mean reducing healthcare costs or becoming more focused and efficient at work to achieve a promotion. Goals and the motivations behind them are as relative and dynamic as the people who set them, so it doesn't matter if your objective is extrinsic or intrinsic. What matters is that the goal is powerful to you.

Overcoming Bad Habits and Bad Times

Our motivation for weight-loss success can often be derailed by bad habits or life's unexpected curveballs. When things are stable, we're able to fast successfully and be mindful of our sugar intake. When life is chaotic, we tend to fall back into our deeply ingrained old dietary habits.

This is why it's so important for me to understand what is motivating a client to make a change. If someone is trying to improve their health so they can be around to see their grandchildren grow up, for example, that motivation is a great way for me to help them stay inspired or get back on track. If that client reports having a lot of energy while they were babysitting their grandkids, I remind them of their motivation and help them create positive associations with fasting and their goal.

Easy Ways to Motivate Yourself

- Go online and read testimonials from people who have reached their weight-loss and health goals through fasting.

- Listen to relevant podcasts and save the most motivating ones for review when you need an extra kick.

- Read books about fasting and write down pages that inspire you for future reference.

- Carry around a note to yourself about why you're doing this, so you can read it when you're tempted to break your fast on a stressful day.

- Keep old blood test results with you to inspire you to stay the course.

Prioritize

One of the biggest struggles I have with clients is that they often have too many goals, and because of that, they want to dive into a fasting program before they've had a chance to prepare for it. For example, they may want to lose 150 pounds, stop taking their medications, reverse their type 2 diabetes, *and* avoid the Alzheimer's diagnosis that runs in their family. These are wonderful goals, but they can't all be achieved at once, no matter how hard you try.

I help clients prioritize their goals by asking two questions: "What is going to kill you first?" and "How strong is your fasting muscle?" Most are aware that they need to lose weight in order to reverse their type 2 diabetes, which will result in a reduction in the number of medications they take every day. If they don't beat that, they're putting themselves at high risk for metabolic-related cancers and Alzheimer's disease. Therefore, diabetes is a disease that may kill them first, and it's what they need to focus on first and foremost.

But these eager clients can't and shouldn't dive into something as intense as an all-day fast. Many of them haven't fasted longer than twelve hours for a blood test before, so fasting for twenty-four hours straight, right off the bat, isn't going to be an easy task. With priorities, you can focus, which may help an impatient person proceed to fast slowly. For example, you may choose to skip breakfast two nonconsecutive days a week, then increase the frequency bit by bit.

As Eve said, I encourage you to write down a list of your goals and prioritize them. The most successful people concentrate on one thing at a time, and they know that trying to do too much at once will inevitably lead to failure. You don't want to take chances on your health, so be patient and consistent. If you are, you *will* reach your goals.

PART 5

DESIGNING YOUR OWN INTERMITTENT FASTING

Common Questions About Fasting

When you start fasting, you're likely to have a lot of questions. We'll discuss many of those issues in <u>Part IV</u> of the book, but we want to address here a few of the most common questions we receive from clients and readers.

Do I have to practice extended fasting for long-term success?

It depends on your fasting goals.

How much weight will I lose when fasting?

Not including water weight, you'll lose about half a pound of body fat per twenty-four hours of fasting. Men and women lose weight at different rates, however. See <u>here</u> for details.

What is the difference between fasting and starving?

Starvation is not voluntary; fasting is. Most people who fast are not malnourished individuals. They tend to be overweight and overnourished.

How long do I have to fast to get into a fat-burning mode?

It begins after having fasted for sixteen hours straight. If you fast just by skipping lunch, you're certainly working your fasting muscle, but you're not yet in the fat-burning zone.

What is autophagy, and when does it start?

The word *autophagy* derives from the Greek "auto" (self) and "phagein" (to eat). The word literally means "to eat oneself." This is the body's way of getting rid of all the broken-down, old cell parts that don't serve the body. It's different for everyone, but it starts after twenty-four to thirty-six hours of not eating, increases 300 percent at thirty-six hours, and plateaus at seventy-two hours. The study of autophagy is relatively new, and, as such, our knowledge of it is incomplete. Thus, it's recommended if you are fasting for autophagy that you only consume water and salt.

I've heard that fasting can burn muscle. Is this true?

Up to about twenty-four hours or so during a fast, the body mostly uses glucose for energy. During the switch from burning glucose to burning fat, there is a short period when the body uses protein to produce new glucose for energy. This phase is called gluconeogenesis. Many people assume that this period of burning protein is detrimental to health, but it's likely the opposite. Protein is not the same as muscle, so burning protein does not necessarily mean that you are burning muscle. You also have lots of skin and connective tissue. During longer fasts, the body switches to burning mostly fat for energy, and this period of protein metabolism stops.

Can I work out while fasting?

Yes! Movement is encouraged while fasting. When you feel lethargic on a fast, the worst thing you can do is do nothing. Walking is great. Vertical movements aid weight loss because they drain the lymphatic system. Some individuals prefer to work out in a fasted state, and professional athletes sometimes train in a fasted state.

I'm afraid that if I fast, I will just overeat later and gain weight. Does that happen?

No. Most people report a dramatic decrease in appetite. Mentally, they may feel hungry, but as soon as they start to eat, they fill up quite quickly.

Will I lose hair from fasting?

Hair loss is one of the people's biggest fears because they think that if their hair is falling out, they must be malnourished, but that's not the case. Hair loss is not associated with fasting; it is associated with rapid weight loss. Those who practice intermittent fasting and lose weight steadily—rather than rapidly—don't have issues, as their body is expecting weight loss. Those who do extended fasts or experience a drastic change in body composition experience hair loss regardless of the type of diet they're on. Hair loss can be stopped by slowing down weight loss, or you can wait it out once the rapid weight loss is over.

Will I have extra skin when I lose weight?

It depends on the individual. Our program has yet to have one client require skin removal surgery since we started in 2012.

How much water should I have daily?

How much water you need varies from person to person, so you should drink water whenever you're thirsty. Thirst is also frequently mistaken for hunger, so drink when you feel hungry, too.

How much salt should I consume daily?

It completely varies per person. Start with $^1/4$ teaspoon in your water and continue to add more until you stop experiencing headaches or lethargy.

Can I drink alcohol while fasting?

We don't suggest it. Alcohol puts you at risk for dehydration and can raise your insulin levels, which you're trying to lower during a fast. We even recommend abstaining from alcohol—except, if you wish, a glass of wine—during your first meal after a fast. If you do drink, I recommend dry wines (red or white) and spirits as long as the mixers don't have sugars or sweeteners in them. For example, a vodka soda with lime won't raise your insulin-like, say, a margarita. Also, we encourage people to limit themselves to one drink per day. If you drink more than one alcoholic beverage, alternate the booze with a glass of water. Finally, it's better to consume alcohol during rather than outside your eating windows (say, during the time you've set aside for dinner).

Can I have sugar or stevia while fasting?

This is a hard no. Both sugar and stevia will stimulate the production of insulin, which you are trying to reduce with fasting.

Can I take my vitamin or daily supplements while fasting?

Supplements may hinder autophagy. When fasting for metabolic reasons (meaning insulin resistance-related conditions such as type 2 diabetes, obesity, PCOS, and nonalcoholic fatty liver disease), the effectiveness of supplements is questionable. Most vitamins are fat-soluble, but if you're not taking in fat, they won't be as effective. Probiotics are fine to continue taking while fasting.

What do I do about medications I normally take with food?

Talk to your doctor.

Step One: How Not to Snack

The rules are simple. Eat three meals a day until you are full. Each meal should take no longer than one hour, and you get to choose the time of the meals. You get to pick the food in the meals. If you drink soda or any kind of drink, even diet drinks, start limiting them to your mealtimes. If you must have gum, have it after you eat and within one hour of a meal. But, *no snacks*, which means: no gum, candy, mints, sugar, food, juice, sweet drinks— natural or otherwise—broth, smoothies, or sports drinks, except at mealtimes.

If this sounds easy to you, then I completely admire you. And, pardon the pun, but I bet fasting might just end up being a piece of cake for you. If you're a bit older, like myself, not snacking may even sound familiar. I remember being told that if I had a snack after school, it would spoil my dinner. Eventually, the prevailing wisdom changed, and parents—mine included—gave their children snacks after school.

Baby Steps May Be Necessary

Some of you reading this may realize that you eat eight to ten times a day. If that's the case, don't stop snacking cold turkey. If you do, you'd be eating only a third of the times that you currently do. This compares to a person smoking a pack of cigarettes a day going to just a few cigarettes a day. You're likely to fail quickly, and I don't want that to happen. Instead, cut out one snack time per day for a week, just like this:

- **WEEK 1**: Go from eating eight times a day to eating seven times a day.

- **WEEK 2**: Go from eating seven times a day to eating six times a day.

- **WEEK 3**: Go from eating six times a day to eating five times a day.

Get the picture?

When I stopped snacking, it was uncomfortable, but it was not painful or unbearable. It just felt foreign because I was used to eating at certain times of the day, and my body and mind knew it. At first, I felt hungry during the periods I would usually eat. But my body began to adjust, and I didn't expect the food I had been giving it at that time slot. When I skipped my usual snack, I also felt hungrier than normal at my next eating period, and I would eat a bit extra then. But my body adjusted to this over time, too.

I now avoid snacking about 90 percent of the time, and it's one of the reasons I feel that I've been able to maintain a healthier weight for the first time in my life. Sometimes, I can't resist sneaking in something extra delicious, or if I have a hunger that lasts for hours, I may have a snack. But this is rare. Thankfully, now that I'm used to it, staying away from snacks isn't as hard as I thought it would be. I understand that fit people do the right things *most* of the time, and that is what I strive for.

Step Two: Skip Breakfast

Yep, that's it. Instead of eating three meals a day, you will eat two. And remember, no snacks.

How can you prepare the night before you skip breakfast? Great question. Your dinner should consist of healthy, whole foods that will fill you up and make you feel good. Preferably, stick to a low-carb diet. When you eat sugary foods or other products you've decided are not great for you, they can make you feel hungrier the next morning. I find it helpful to consume lots of healthy fat the night before fasting, like meat or cheese, plus a big green salad loaded with vegetables. You should eat this meal within one hour, a time period that allows you to enjoy what you're eating and who you're eating with—and get full.

When you skip breakfast the next day, you will be hungry at first because your body is used to eating in the morning. Distract yourself by hydrating instead. Drink water, carbonated water, tea, or coffee. If you must, have a splash of heavy cream in your tea or coffee. I skip breakfast every morning, but I drink two cups of coffee, and they set me right. Do not use sugar or sweetener of any kind, including natural sweeteners like stevia. Why? Because for many people, that sweetness can very well trigger hunger and make fasting more difficult than it needs to be. Remember, weight loss is about controlling hunger, not calories. When it's time for lunch, eat within your one-hour eating period, then wait no more than eight hours until dinner, when you should dine within one hour again.

There was a time when I woke up and ate as soon as possible, hoping to get my metabolism running. Now, I rarely eat in the morning, and it has come to be no big deal. In fact, I was shocked to find that once I was used to it—which took me about six months—I hardly ever felt hungry. If I did, my trusty coffee with a splash of heavy cream did the trick.

How often you choose to skip breakfast is completely up to you. Suppose the first day feels like no big deal; skip breakfast again the next day. If not eating is hell, only do it once or twice a week until it is bearable. Eventually, step up your frequency (I recommend adding one day a week, day by day) until you reach a place that's comfortable for you.

You may have an unusual schedule and want to know if you can skip dinner instead of breakfast. Of course, you can! The meal you choose not to eat doesn't matter. The goal here is for you to get comfortable with eating only two meals a day, each consumed within one hour, separated by no more than eight hours between the two meals.

Can you still work out on the morning that you fast? Yes, you certainly can. I do, and I find I exercise so much better while I'm fasting than I do when I work out after eating. Another unexpected surprise for me about skipping breakfast is that now my family has more time to sit together on the sofa, sip coffee, and give the doggy extra belly rubs. Plus, we don't have to do breakfast dishes before we run out the door, and we save money on groceries. Win-win!

In short, skip breakfast as frequently as you wish and see what changes happen in your body and mind. I know many people who do this daily, and this is the total extent of their fasting practice. I've seen these people lose weight, get off medications, and change their lives for the better. This may be the case for you, or you may find after a time that you wish to go further. Again, it's up to you. This is *your* life.

Step Three: Skip Lunch

Now that you are never snacking and regularly and comfortably skipping breakfast as often as you wish, you're ready for a day where you only eat an evening meal.

If you think about it, skipping lunch after not eating breakfast only adds about six more hours of fasting. For most people, it also isn't nearly as traumatizing as they think it will be. Plus, you only have to *try* for *one day*. The following day, you can go back to the eating schedule you normally follow.

Yes, you are going to get hungry at lunchtime, but keep yourself busy, hydrated, distracted, and determined to reach your goals. When dinnertime rolls around, eat healthy, filling foods for a period of one hour, and make sure to finish up at least two hours before you go to bed.

If eating the only dinner for a day isn't that difficult, try it again the following week. If the process continues to be easy for you, begin eating the only dinner two days per week but not on consecutive days. After a period of time you feel comfortable with, decide if you want to eat the only dinner three days a week, nonconsecutively.

Does it matter which meals you skip? Just as with step one, no. You can eat at the mealtime of your choosing. I have suggested eating only at dinner because this is the meal most commonly shared by family or socially. If you have an untraditional schedule, feel free to go with just breakfast, or you could choose to eat only lunch. The only necessity is that you eat a meal with a fasting period of twenty-three hours before it. So, if you decide to eat only lunch, your last meal the day before would need to be lunch.

As a person who had zero experience fasting before I dove into this new lifestyle, I never found a twenty-four-hour fast too mentally or physically difficult. I'd worked up to it by skipping snacks and breakfast, so one more meal didn't seem terrible. I still feel this way, and now I skip breakfast most days.

Tracking Your Fasting

Over the years, I've seen many people track their twenty-four-hour fasts using a timer or an app. They find it's not only helpful but gives them a feeling of accomplishment to see the hours they've fasted climbing—from fourteen to eighteen to . . . time's up! Dinner's ready! If this helps you, go for it! Personally, I found tracking my fasting hours, not to be helpful. I began to focus on how long I had left and then dwelled on the fact that my belly was empty. It caused me to doubt if I could finish the fast, and I realized that the busier and more distracted I became, the better I could enjoy the process. But you may be different!

Step Four: Skip Dinner

I'm going, being honest; I think that step four is the most difficult. But if you have stopped snacking, often skip breakfast, and are at ease with bypassing lunch a few times a week— yet still aren't hitting your weight loss and health goals—then it is time for a thirty-six-hour fast.

I know, I know! You may be thinking, *Wait. Thirty-six hours? I thought I was only fasting for a full day?* Stop for a second and think: This fast is referred to as a 36 because you will not be eating for thirty-six hours. You finish dinner at, say, 7:00 p.m. You sleep for the night. You don't eat the following day. You sleep again. You wake up and eat breakfast at 7 a.m. Boom, you just fasted for thirty-six hours!

I didn't use the schedule above for my first thirty-six-hour fast, and I found it extremely difficult. Why? Because I was awake for a lot more of it, obsessing over my hunger. I ate breakfast and then began a thirty-six-hour fast, which means I was only asleep for eight hours of it. It is *so* much easier to do a thirty-six-hour fast when you are asleep for sixteen hours of fasting time. This means you only deal with hunger for twenty hours or the hours that you are awake.

I recommend scheduling this fast on a day you are as busy as possible and around as little food as possible. Set yourself up for success, not suffering, and do your best to limit mealtimes with others, shopping, and cooking. Because these things are sometimes unavoidable, you should always ask for support, and you may just be surprised at how helpful people will be. I also tend to sleep less when I fast for a full day, and while this was once confusing and discouraging, I now view it as an opportunity, and I plan to get extra things done when I'm not sleeping.

Finally, remember that not eating for one day is called *fasting*, not *starving*. The choice is the differentiator, and while going to bed with no food in your stomach may be scary, once you're asleep, you won't even notice. Plus, during the day, you can practice all the tricks you did before: hydrate, find an activity you enjoy and remind yourself that you're doing awesome things to reach your goal.

Will you be hungry? Yes! You aren't used to going a day without food, and your body is going to get hungry in response to the behaviors it has been used to. But remember that hunger isn't a bad thing; it's your body telling you it's burning fat. Plus, you're heading into uncharted territory here, and every time you fast is a singular experience. When you lengthen a fast for a longer period than you have ever done before, you will probably feel hungrier. But you can handle it because you've built up to it.

The frequency of a thirty-six-hour fast is completely up to you. If you find your first 36 traumatic, wait one month before trying it again. If you think it's pretty darn easy, do it again the following week. As the thirty-six-hour fast becomes more seamless, you can use it as a tool to speed up your progress toward your goals.

Tips for Getting to Sleep After a Full Day of Fasting

1. Remind yourself that the sooner you get to sleep, the sooner you will eat in the morning.

2. Make sure you are well hydrated. Some people find a mug of warm caffeine-free tea (like chamomile) helps them to feel fuller.

3. Consider melatonin supplements if needed.

4. Warm baths are great but are most helpful at least a few hours before bedtime.

5. Avoid computer, TV, and phone screens for a couple of hours before bed if possible.

6. Try meditating, deep breathing, aromatherapy, reading, or whatever makes you feel restful.

7.   Decide what you will eat for breakfast. Don't prepare it because you might end up shoving some of it into your mouth accidentally that night (it has happened to me!). Knowing what you are looking forward to enjoying foodwise in the morning can make hunger more bearable.

Step Five: Extend the Fast to Day Two

Just look at you! You have become an impressive fasting beast. You stopped snacking, often skip breakfast, can also skip lunch when you choose, and can even go a full day with no food. Guess what? You've already completed an extended fast because most people define one as being longer than twenty-four hours. Nice going!

So how does one prepare to not eat for *more* than one day? First, you must decide if you want to do it at all. So many people have lost weight and met all their health goals without ever doing an extended fast, and that is more than fine. For example, one woman I followed online stopped snacking, and skipped breakfast every morning. With this schedule, she lost sixty pounds in a year, and her doctor took her off her medication for type 2 diabetes because her blood sugars were in a healthy range. Another man I followed lost over one hundred pounds over a nine-month period by skipping breakfast every day and forgoing lunch on two of those days. He also lowered his blood pressure and was taken off the medication he had used for eighteen years.

This is not the case for everyone, though, and there are many reasons you might want to try an extended fast. They include:

- You want to speed up the process toward your goal.
- Your weight and measurements have stalled for a month or more.
- You are curious to see what it is like.
- You are seeking added health benefits beyond just weight loss. For example, extended fasts are more effective at lower insulin levels in those with type 2 diabetics. After thirty-six hours, ketosis begins, and after forty-eight hours, autophagy, or the process of cellular cleansing, kick-starts. Extended fasts are also reported to heighten mental clarity.

To strengthen your fasting muscles and see if an extended fast will work for you, start by not eating for a whole day, sleeping, and then fasting until lunch the following day. If this feels comfortable, a few days or so later, try forty-two hours. Then forty-eight. Later, step up to seventy-two hours, then five days. The important thing is to increase your fasting window bit by bit. Once one fasting regimen becomes easy, then extend it to the next level of fasting.

It is tempting to think that the longer the fast, the better. This simply isn't the case. I have done two extremely long fasts: one for eleven days and one for ten days. My results were impressive: I lost about twelve pounds each time, and my skin glowed like I'd had a $300 facial at a fancy spa. But the fasting was very tough mentally, and my weight loss was the same as it would have been if I'd just fasted for ten single, nonconsecutive days over a month. Other than those, I have done about twenty extended fasts, most being thirty-six to forty-eight hours. They can be tough for me to stick to, but if I schedule them when I am busy and when my husband can cook and grocery shop, I can usually complete them.

How do you exercise while fasting?

- **CHOOSE SOMETHING YOU CAN AFFORD, AND THAT FITS IN YOUR SCHEDULE.** Don't sign up for a marathon if you can only devote two hours a week to running. Don't enroll inexpensive private Pilates classes that your budget will not allow.

- **FIND SOMETHING THAT YOU ENJOY.** If you are groaning now, I get it. I used to hate any and all kinds of exercise because getting up and moving was painful. I chose walking because I enjoyed the peace of being outside, and I worked my way into it slowly. If you can't find an exercise you like right away, then choose to exercise in an environment you enjoy. For example, if you're looking for a low-impact way to reduce stress, try gentle yoga. If you love the pool, sign up for a water aerobics class.

- **CONSIDER DOING LESS CARDIO AND MORE STRENGTH TRAINING.** Many people who haven't found a great exercise routine find cardio intimidating because it wears them out quickly. You can work your way into strength training slowly and build up. Seeing progress as you add more and more weights to your routine is *so* satisfying.

- **ONCE YOUR EXERCISE ROUTINE BECOMES EASY OR BORING, ADD SOMETHING TO IT, MAKE IT MORE DIFFICULT, OR CHANGE THE ENVIRONMENT.** Your body is highly adaptable, and without constant change, your workouts will decrease ineffectiveness.

- **EXAMINE YOUR MOOD EACH WEEK AND LOOK FOR A CONNECTION BETWEEN YOUR WORKOUTS AND YOUR MENTAL STATE.** Do you feel calmer when you take walks outside? Do you feel happier when you lift weights a few times a week? Many people find that exercise is a huge influence on their emotional state.

- **GET AN EXERCISE BUDDY.** Exercise is a great excuse to spend time productively with someone you enjoy. This could be your spouse, partner, friend, boss, mom, or neighbor. It really doesn't matter. If you are both fasting, this will also help to replace some of the bonding time you may have spent together in the past eating.

- **OPTIMIZE YOUR WORKOUTS.** Compare your workouts when fasting and feasting to find the ideal time to do them. I personally have a much better workout when I fast, but some people may see better results when feasting.

PART 6

FEASTING WHILE DOING INTERMITTENT FASTING

The truth is we *deserve* to eat, and we *deserve* to enjoy it. I'll admit that changing what I ate was difficult, and giving up sugar felt like a mourning process to me. But by eating the way I have chosen for myself, I am able to eat something outside my healthy food list 10 percent of the time and still maintain my weight loss.

Your friends and family may also be happy and relieved to see you feasting. Although they'll learn to live with your fasting lifestyle, there are times you're going to complain about being hungry or missing foods that are awful for you (Cheetos, anyone?). When you are fasting, remember that it is your choice to do so, and you can end it at any time. This also means you can complain every once in a while—but never forget that it can get annoying for others. After you have fasted, loved ones are going to *want* to see your feast. They need to know you aren't starving yourself and that you have a healthy attitude about nourishing your body. The best way to prove that to them is to enjoy eating food authentically.

So, feast away. Eat delicious food. Enjoy every bite. Munch on healthy, beautiful, delicious morsels and relish every moment of it. People often say that absence makes the heart grow fonder, and that's true for the mouth, too. Fasting can actually heighten your enjoyment of food!

Eating is a natural human process necessary for the continuation of life. Eating should be a joyful experience. Learning to enjoy food without guilt is a powerful step in learning how to fast.

How to Feast without Guilt

1. Gain control of what, when, where, and for how long you will eat. One hour is an ideal amount of time for eating a meal.

2. Remove distractions from your meal. For example, put away your phone, turn off the TV, and put down the book.

3. Remind yourself that you are a living being who is powered by food and that receiving that food is meant to be an enjoyable experience.

4. Eat until you feel comfortably full. Don't stop eating until you have had enough, and don't keep eating because you fear hunger later. There will be an opportunity for more food later.

5. Don't compare your food choices and amounts to others'. Each body is unique.

6. Remember that eating is okay. Do not punish yourself for enjoying food. You deserve nourishment no matter your size. It simply isn't natural for humans to loathe doing something they must do to keep themselves alive.

Five Ways to Feast Responsibly

1. **PLAN AHEAD**: If you have a holiday or vacation coming up, try to fit in a few fasts before and after the event. These can be short or extended fasts depending on how strong your fasting muscle is. But try to stretch a little. If you're someone who usually fasts for twenty-four hours, try to fast for thirty-six hours a week before and after.

2. **TIME YOUR FEAST**: It's better to eat an early dinner rather than a late one because you have a few hours before bedtime to burn off whatever you ate. If you're going to eat carbs or sugar, try to do it midday rather than in the evening or nighttime.

3. **STICK TO A SCHEDULE AND DON'T SNACK**: Enjoy your feast while you're doing it and try not to snack before or after it. Sticking within your meal windows is important because it limits the number of times per day, your body secretes the fat-storing hormone, insulin.

4. **SKIP THE SODAS**: Try to avoid drinking sugary drinks, especially if you know you're going to be indulging in carbs or dessert at a later meal. Be

mindful of what you're mixing your spirits with, too. Margaritas, piña coladas, and many other tropical drinks are extremely sugary, so, if you like mixed drinks, mix the alcohol of your choice with seltzer or soda water and a splash of lime juice instead.

5.   **BE MINDFUL ABOUT WINE**: If you're going to drink wine, try to drink a dry wine, which is a wine with no residual sugar. Unlike Moscato and Riesling, which have higher sugar content, cabernets and dry champagne tend to be lower in sugar, so they are a safe choice if you're staring at a wine list and unsure of what to order.

PART 6

SHORT-LIVED SIDE EFFECTS OF INTERMITTENT FASTING

Bad Breath or Bad Taste in Your Mouth

People sometimes report a metallic taste in their mouth when they start fasting. Others report that their breath smells like nail polish or fruit. This is a sign that your body has entered ketosis. Ketones—beta-hydroxybutyrate, acetoacetate, and acetone—are expelled through urine and exhalation, and they may have an odor (for instance, acetone is one of the ingredients in nail polish). This odor or taste will go away over time, though you may need to brush your teeth more often for the first few weeks.

Bloating

If you're bloated, you may have consumed too much salt, and your body is retaining water because of it. Try reducing your salt intake or drinking water rather than bone broth or another salty beverage.

Coldness

If you feel cold while fasting, that's a sign that your body is entering ketosis. Your body is simply having a bit of trouble moving from burning glucose to burning adequate fat to keep you warm. It's nothing to be concerned about. You should warm up once your body becomes fat-adapted and fully makes the switch from burning sugar to burning fat.

Constipation

Fasting causes your insulin levels to drop, which sends a signal to your kidneys to release stored water. This can cause you to become dehydrated, then constipated. During the days that you aren't fasting, increase the number of leafy greens and fiber you consume. During your fast, soak in Epsom salt baths and take magnesium citrate (at a starting dose of 400 mg once per day) if you must. Hydrate with salt and water.

Many people assume they're constipated during an extended fast when, in fact, they just don't have anything in their intestines. If you haven't had a bowel movement during a long fast, but you aren't cramping, then you're fine.

Depression

People often report feeling less anxious and experiencing an improved mood when they fast. Depression is unusual, so if you do feel depressed, we suggest seeking the advice of a therapist.

Diarrhea

If you experience diarrhea while fasting, try mixing 1 to 2 tablespoons of chia seeds or psyllium husk with water, wait 10 minutes, and drink the mixture. Chia and psyllium both absorb excess water in the digestive tract, allowing less liquid to be expelled with loose stools.

Dizziness

Dizziness is often a sign of mild dehydration. Be sure you're drinking water throughout the day. Consume extra salt in the form of pickle juice or bone broth. Some people, like Eve's dad, may also be experiencing a stabilization of their previously high blood pressure. If you're on blood pressure medication, have started fasting, and are experiencing dizziness, be sure to see your doctor. You may need to lower your medication dosage.

Dry Lips

This may sound counterintuitive, but dry lips are a sign you are drinking too much water and not enough salt. Add salt to your diet in the form of pickle juice or bone broth.

Fatigue

When you start fasting, you may feel tired at first as your body transitions from burning sugar to burning fat. This should pass within your first three or four fasts when you begin to feel more energetic.

Headaches

Headaches are very common when you're fasting. We don't exactly know why they happen, but there is speculation that they may be due to a salt deficiency. To prevent and treat headaches, consume more salt in the form of bone broth or pickle juice. Stay away from ibuprofen and other painkillers.

Heartburn

If there's no food in your belly to absorb your stomach acid, some of it may come up, causing a tight, burning sensation in your chest. Try an over-the-counter antacid or speak to your doctor about a prescription if the problem persists.

Intense Emotions

Volatility and feeling intense, often explosive emotions aren't incredibly common, but they may happen when you start fasting. It's a dramatically new lifestyle, and it's normal for your mind to feel overwhelmed. Hang in there! Surround yourself with people who love and understand you, and seek professional therapy if needed.

Nausea

Feeling nauseated is not considered normal while you're fasting, and it can be a sign of dehydration. Drink water, and if you experience anything more than short bursts of nausea, or if nausea increases to the degree that makes you uncomfortable, stop fasting.

Sleeplessness

Most people report having sleep issues during their first two weeks of intermittent fasting. This is the result of your body adapting to the increased level of adrenaline that it produces while you fast. Create a calming, relaxing bedtime ritual to try to wind down. You might dim the lights, drink a cup of warm herbal tea, and curl up with a book until your body tells you it's ready to sleep. Avoid looking at screens—televisions, phones, laptops, tablets—before bed, as they emit blue light that interferes with sleep. If sleeplessness persists, try taking a melatonin supplement.

Thirst

Increased thirst is completely normal while you're fasting because after your body burns the fuel in your stomach, it burns glycogen. Glycogen is bound with water molecules. Ever hear someone say that, instead of losing fat, you've lost water weight? That's what they're referring to. If you feel thirsty while you're fasting, drink more water. Strive to consume at least half your body weight in pounds to ounces and drink that each day.

Upset Stomach

An upset stomach—as opposed to nausea—is likely just the result of hunger pangs, which can be alleviated by drinking mineral water.

PART 7

HOW TO KEEP INTERMITTENT FASTING GOING FOR LONG TERM?

Forty Things to Do Instead of Eating

When you're fasting and bored, you don't have to do something strenuous, brain-busting, or taxing to fill up your time. You can pick from any of these activities, which will help the minutes (and maybe hours!) fly by.

1. Drink water.
2. Listen to music.
3. Call your mom.
4. Research your next vacation.
5. Go for a walk outside.
6. Clean the kitchen.
7. Walk your dog.
8. Read a book.
9. Update your résumé.
10. Call a friend.
11. Visit the library.
12. Knit or crochet.
13. Journal.
14. Watch a TV show you've never seen before.
15. Do ten jumping jacks.
16. Make a cup of tea.
17. Fold laundry and put it away.
18. Go to a yoga class.
19. Go shopping.
20. Clean out your email inbox.
21. Visit a neighbor.
22. Drop off the dry cleaning.

23.   Say a prayer or meditate.

24.   Organize a closet.

25.   Sit outside in the sun.

26.   Take your child on a fun adventure.

27.   Organize your digital photos.

28.   Scrapbook.

29.   Play a board game.

30.   Listen to an audiobook.

31.   Garden.

32.   Make a craft project.

33.   Go to a museum.

34.   Write a thank-you note.

35.   Read a magazine or newspaper.

36.   Tackle the junk drawer.

37.   Watch old family movies.

38.   Clean the bathroom.

39.   Pick wildflowers and put them in a vase.

40.   Rake or sweep outside.

Things Not to Do While Fasting

There are so many activities that you might not *think* are centered on food, but in fact, highlight food prominently. If you participate in them while you're fasting, I can promise you you'll start doing mental somersaults around the idea of eating, and before you know it, your hand will be in the cookie jar.

I'm warning you! From the moment you begin a fast to the minute you end it, you should avoid the following activities:

Looking at Social Media

Guess what people post on social media? Pictures of delicious-looking food! If you are like me, when you are first learning to fast, it's impossible to resist running to the refrigerator when images of food pop up every two seconds. Worse than the temptation, though, is the self-loathing you might feel. I've found myself getting frustrated looking at these photos and associating them with the person who posted the images. I start to think, *How can [this person] eat all this sugar and fried food and look so great? Why am I the only person who can't have food?*

Of course, these are ridiculous statements, but they eat away at you at a time when you need to be strong and confident. Remember, you are in control. You are the person who has made the decision to get healthy. You are the one who has decided to fast, and *you* can stop fasting at absolutely any moment.

Grocery Shopping

Fasting helped me become a better grocery shopper and a better cook. If I was going to eat fewer times, then I was going to make sure the meals I did prepare were delicious and enjoyable.

When I'm fasting, though, I can't grocery shop. Even if I'm not hungry, I start battling with my reflexes any time I see a free food sample in the grocery store. As I push my shopping cart down the aisles, I feel like I am surrounded by temptation and things I can't have. I become so resentful and deprived that I usually break my fast sooner than I want to. Sometimes, I go on to eat more than I truly need.

I strongly recommend planning your grocery shopping carefully before or after your fast, even if you are feeding a family. Ask for help from family members or use a delivery service if possible.

Cooking

When I am fasting, I do not cook. The sight, feel, and smell of food is too much for my senses to overcome. This is not about my lack of willpower, either. When your senses are bombarded by food, it's only natural for you to want to taste it.

Not everyone is in this position, though, so if you have to cook while you're fasting, here are a few tips I recommend:

- Prep your family's meals before your fast so you can just heat things up.
- Ask for help from family members who are able to cook.
- Buy prepared foods or send your family out to eat.
- Cook items that are their favorites but aren't yours.
- Turn on the vent or open the window to reduce the smell of food.

Cleaning Dishes

You might be surprised to hear this, but cleaning dishes for others is tough for me when I am fasting. Years ago, I "accidentally" stuck my finger in the leftover pudding and licked it, and once a piece of chicken on a dirty plate ended up in my mouth on hour forty-two of a forty-eight-hour fast. I had decades of experience snacking and nibbling, and breaking this bad habit took time.

Now, I am much more accustomed to fasting, so I could probably wash dirty dishes with ease while I'm not eating.

Going to the Mall

Going shopping at the local mall seemed like a great idea when I first started fasting. After all, what was I supposed to do with all that extra time on my hands? Indulge in a little retail therapy! But when I stepped into the mall, the smell from the pretzel shop wafted out and slapped me across the face. I felt angry at the people walking around holding cinnamon rolls and pizza slices, and I wondered if I could just maybe have a bite or two.

Today, I can go to the mall with ease while fasting and still love my fellow humans—even when they have a giant pretzel. But that wasn't the case at first, so don't make the same mistake I did.

Going to the Movies

I love going to the movies. It used to mean a cool, safe place to shove all the popcorn and candy into my face in the dark without the judgment of others. As I changed my eating, I switched the popcorn and Coke out for a giant dill pickle and water, and I felt pretty happy. But, even today, the idea of fasting at the movies just does not sound fun to me. I know I should be well adjusted to fasting and at the theater only for the entertainment, but, unfortunately, I can't break the habit of wanting to eat in a theater. You may feel the same.

I suggest you remove yourself from the situation and plan your movie theater outings for when you're feasting. You can watch plenty of movies at home without needing to snack.

Going to a Party

I plan my fasting around social events. There is a time to fast, and there is a time to feast, and, for me, a party is a time to feast.

As a middle-aged married woman with a preteen, I realize that my social life isn't filled with fancy, food-centric soirees all the time, so this is easier for me. If your lifestyle requires frequent social gatherings, and you can't schedule your fasts around them, try holding a glass of water or a club soda with lime in your hand while you're working the room. People will question you less about eating, and having a glass to carry will give you something to do. In addition, waiters will offer you food less often if you are drinking and socializing. You may think people watch everything you eat, but often they won't even notice if you go to a party, have a few cleverly disguised drinks, socialize all night, and eat nothing. If they do offer you something to eat, the easiest thing to do is to thank them and say you aren't hungry at the moment.

Going on Vacation

I am comfortable with intermittent fasting on vacation, but extended fasting is tough for me if I'm away from home. I like to experience different cultures and places through food, so a long fast while I'm on a trip, makes me feel like I'm losing opportunities to learn something. However, intermittent fasting on vacation works great for me because I feel like I can make one or two meals that day really count with a feast.

This list of dos and don'ts while fasting may be different for everyone. Like anything else, fasting truly gets easier with practice. I honestly didn't believe that when I started, but it is true. At first, I couldn't go to parties, the mall, or near any store with food while fasting. Now, I can do most of these things with ease. Just remember: You get to make the decisions of when you will fast and when you will stop. You get to be in control. You get to decide what is best for your mind and body during this entire process. For control freaks like me, once you accept that you are truly in charge, fasting becomes an enjoyable thing to do.

Finally, don't judge yourself so harshly if you need special circumstances when you first start fasting. I made that mistake and saw myself as weak.

I wasn't weak, I was inexperienced, and I got more experienced over time.

Now, I know I am strong. I gave myself the time and situations to develop the skill of fasting. I am not the secret loser I thought I was! You deserve to give yourself the best chance of success. And bit by bit, you'll see your body and your mind begin to change into what you always dreamed they could be.

How to Deal with Nosy Friends, Co-workers, and Partygoers

When I began fasting, I was surprised by the reactions and opinions of the people around me—at the office, at home, at parties, or just in everyday life when I chose not to eat. A lot of people didn't notice, but some did, and they had no problem sharing their views. These people had been used to me eating all the time, and they were confused when I passed on the candy jar, the birthday cupcakes, or the afternoon chips. At first, some *insisted* that I have a snack. Once they got used to my responses to snacks, though, they offered less, and not snacking got a bit easier for me.

If you're presented with something to eat, try saying:

- "No, thanks, I'm full."
- "Thank you, but I'm not hungry."
- "It looks great, but I already ate."
- "I'm good for now."
- "It looks great, but I'm all set."
- "I may check it out later, but right now, I don't feel like eating."

Try *not* to say:

- "I'm fasting."
- "I'm not snacking anymore."
- "I do not eat snacks."

If you do, you're opening yourself up for a big discussion (or confrontation!), and the well-intentioned snack bearers may feel that they need to defend their choice to nibble. Unless you're with your most trusted friends or loved ones, it's often easier to avoid the conversation entirely.

Adjust Your Priorities

Fasting is going to require that you alter some things yourself and how you spend your time. After all, if you changed nothing about your life, you would end up living in the exact same body you decided could use some improvement. If your social life consists of business lunches five days a week, happy hours with appetizers five days a week, weekend brunches with friends, Friday night dinners with your spouse, and Sunday all-day eating with your family, then yes, you are going to have to make major changes to your social life. You are going to have to adjust your priorities and choose to fast over a life that revolves around food. Luckily, if you're like me, you can look at your schedule and realize there are minor alterations you can make that will deliver big results.

Know Your Limits

Many of us put ourselves in truly difficult situations to try to prove we are strong enough. This is a ridiculous and painful way to handle things. What if instead you treated yourself kindly and gave yourself the best possible chance of succeeding?

Now that I know I can fast successfully and have maintained my weight for the first time in my life, I know when fasting is the right choice for me. Personally, I do not fast for longer than seventeen hours at a time while on vacation or when my extended family is visiting because I know, there will be delicious food around that I want to enjoy. I choose to do longer fasts when I am at home, usually just with my husband, and I can keep busy. These are the easiest times for me to be successful.

When do you have the best chances of success? This is when you should schedule your fasting. Fasting is not about saying no to yourself. Fasting is about saying yes to yourself on your own terms!

All these techniques may feel odd at first, but over time they become natural, and you stop noticing that you have to do them. To truly change your mind and body, you must expect to make changes to your environment—but that's not a bad thing. It can be empowering to realize how much of your environment you can control. Give yourself the time you need to adopt the new behaviors and be patient with yourself. Soon, you *will* begin to enjoy your time at home, at work, at the grocery store, and at restaurants more than you would have ever believed possible because there will be fewer decisions and less stress. Notice your successes, even the small ones, and give yourself credit for making each change. These changes add up quickly, and suddenly, there is a new, happier you are staring back from the mirror!

If you feel you have appreciated my effort, I kindly ask you to leave a (positive) review! It will help me to create something new and useful for your interest: =) *M.T.*